THE *Skinny*
SLOW COOKER
RECIPE BOOK

The Skinny Slow Cooker Recipe Book.
Delicious recipes under 300, 400 and 500 calories.

A Bell & Mackenzie Publication
First published in 2013 by Bell & Mackenzie Publishing
Copyright © Bell & Mackenzie Publishing 2013

ISBN 978-0-9576447-8-6

Disclaimer
The information and advice in this book is intended as
a guide only. Any individual should independently seek
the advice of a health professional before embarking
on a diet. Some recipes may contain nuts or traces of
nuts. Those suffering from any allergies associated with
nuts should avoid any recipes containing nuts or nut
based oils.

Contents

Contents

Contents

Skinny
SLOW COOKER
INTRODUCTION

Introduction

Welcome to The Skinny Slow Cooker Recipe Book: Delicious Recipes Under 300, 400 and 500 Calories.

This collection of easy to prepare and delicious low-calorie recipes will help you make inexpensive, healthy meals for you and your family with the minimum of fuss. During the colder 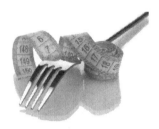 months our bodies naturally crave warm, filling and comforting food which can often result in overeating, weight gain and sluggishness.

These delicious recipes use simple and inexpensive fresh ingredient; are packed full of flavour and goodness, and show that you can enjoy maximum taste with minimum calories.

Each recipe has been tried, tested, and enjoyed time and time again. With so many delicious recipes to choose from, we're sure you'll agree that with 'The Skinny Slow Cooker Recipe Book', *diet* can still mean *delicious*!

Preparation

All of the recipes take no longer than 10-15 minutes to prepare. Browning the meat will make a difference to the taste of your recipe but if you really don't have the time, don't worry. It will still taste good.

There are a number of 'shortcut' ingredients like salsa and taco rub throughout the book, but there is also the option to make these from scratch if you have the time.

All meat and vegetables should be cut into even sized pieces.

Meat generally cooks faster than vegetables, although root vegetables can take longer, so make sure everything is bite-sized.

All meat should be trimmed of visible fat and the skin removed.

Nutrition

All of the recipes in this collection are balanced low fat family meals under 500 calories which should keep you feeling full and help you avoid snacking in-between meals. All recipes have serving suggestions; the calories noted 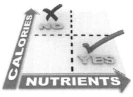 are per serving of the recipe ingredients only, so bear that in mind.

Low Cost

Slow cooking is ideal for cheaper meat cuts. The 'tougher' cuts used in this collection of recipes are transformed into meat which melts-in-your-mouth and helps to keep the costs down. We've also made sure not to include too many one-off ingredients which are used for a single recipe and never used again. All the herbs and spices listed can be used in multiple recipes throughout the book.

Using Your Slow Cooker: A Few Things

All cooking times are a guide. Make sure you get to know your own slow cooker so that you can adjust timings accordingly.

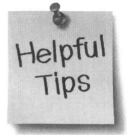

A spray of one cal cooking oil in the cooker before adding ingredients will help with cleaning or you can buy liners.

Be confident with your cooking. Feel free to use substitutes to suit your own taste and don't let a missing herb or spice stop you making a meal - you'll almost always be able to find something to replace it.

Skinny
SLOW COOKER
CHICKEN DISHES

Rustic Chicken Stew
Serves 6

480
CALORIES
PER SERVING

Ingredients:

2kg/4 ½ lb skinless chicken pieces
2 tbsp plain/all purpose flour
1 onion, chopped
1 red (bell) pepper, sliced
2 cloves garlic, crushed
2 400g/14oz tins chopped tomatoes

1 tsp dried rosemary
1 handful pitted green olives
1 tsp anchovy paste
3 bay leaves
500ml/2 cups chicken stock
Low cal cooking spray
Salt & pepper to taste

Method:

Season the chicken pieces well. Dust with the flour and then quickly brown in a large pan with a little low cal cooking spray.

When browned, remove the chicken from the pan and place in the slow cooker with all the other ingredients. Leave to cook on low for 5-6 hours or high for 3-4 hours with the lid tightly shut or until the chicken is cooked through and tender. If you prefer the sauce to be a little thicker, continue cooking for about 45 min on the high setting with the lid removed.

Widely known in Italy as 'Hunter's Stew', this hearty meal has kept the faith with countless hunters and gatherers over the years. Regional 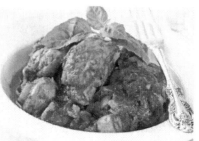 *variations of this dish are common throughout Italy - this rustic version is one of the most popular.*

Sweet Asian Chicken
Serves 4

256
CALORIES
PER SERVING

Ingredients:

500g/1lb 2oz skinless chicken breasts
2 garlic cloves, crushed
1 onion, chopped
60ml/ ¼ cup honey
2 tbsp tomato puree/paste
4 tbsp light soy sauce

2 carrots cut into batons
Pinch crushed chilli
250ml/1 cup fresh orange juice
1 tsp sunflower oil
1 tsp cornstarch dissolved in a little water to form a paste

Method:

Combine all the ingredients in a bowl and add to the slow cooker. Cook on low for 5-6 hours or on high for 3-4 hours with the lid tightly shut or until the chicken is cooked through and tender. Add a little water during cooking if needed.

Serve with fine egg noodles or rice. You could add a garnish of spring onions/scallions & sesame seeds.

The honey, soy and orange juice in this dish make it a hit with the kids and adds a little eastern flavour to evening meal times.

13

Green Pesto Chicken Thighs
Serves 4

469 CALORIES PER SERVING

Ingredients:

500g/1lb 2oz skinless, boneless chicken thighs
175g/6oz green pesto
250ml/1 cup buttermilk

1 tsp salt
50g/2 oz asparagus spears
2 cloves garlic, crushed
1 onion, chopped

Method:

Smother the chicken thighs in pesto and carefully combine with all the other ingredients, except the asparagus spears, in the slow cooker. Cook on low for 5-6 hours or on high for 3-4 hours with the lid tightly shut. Half an hour before cooking ends add the asparagus spears. Ensure the chicken is cooked through and tender. Serve with fresh green salad and crusty bread.

Originating in Northern Italy, pesto has been around since Ancient Roman times. It's pounded blend of basil, cheese, pine nuts, salt and olive oil create a distinctive taste which works well with meat. Pour any juices from the bottom of the slow cooker over the chicken before serving.

Honeyed Chicken Wings

Serves 4

Ingredients:

16 large chicken wings
1 tsp freshly grated ginger (or ½ tsp ground ginger)
2 cloves garlic, crushed
1 tbsp runny honey
1 tbsp light soy sauce
1 tsp sesame oil

1 tbsp lemon juice
1 carrot peeled into ribbons
4 spring onions/scallions chopped
120ml/1/2 cup stock
2 tsp sesame seeds
Salt and pepper to taste

Method:

Coat the chicken wings in the runny honey and then combine with all the other ingredients, except the spring onions and sesame seeds, in the slow cooker. Leave to cook on high for approx 4 hours or low for 6 hours. Serve sprinkled with the spring onions and sesame seeds.

This is a lovely sweet tender chicken recipe which is great to share with family & friends.

Fall Off The Bone Whole Slow Cooked Chicken

446 CALORIES PER SERVING

Serves 6

Ingredients:

2kg/ 4 ½lb whole chicken
2 onions, sliced into rings
Dried rub mix of :
1 tsp each garlic powder,
thyme, paprika & onion powder
+ pinch salt

Method:

Combine the dried ingredients together and rub really well into the fresh chicken.

Place the onions in the bottom of the slow cooker and put the chicken on top. Cook on low for 7-8 hours with the lid tightly shut. Ensure the chicken is cooked through and enjoy the taste of chicken cooked just the way it should be.

Serve with your choice of vegetables, potatoes or salad.

Whole cooked chicken really comes into it's own in the slow cooker. This super simple recipe will give you the heart of a meal which, with leftovers, can last a couple of days.

Zingy Lime Chicken
Serves 4

Ingredients:

500g/1lb 2oz skinless chicken breasts
3 tbsp lime juice
Bunch fresh coriander/cilantro chopped and some to garnish
1 sliced green chilli (or a pinch of dried chilli flakes)
400g/14oz salsa

Or make your own:
Add 1 onion chopped, 1 clove garlic crushed, 1 green chilli chopped to 2 x 400g/14oz tins chopped tomatoes + sea salt to taste
4 tsp your favourite packet taco seasoning

Or make your own:
2 tsp mild chilli powder, 1 ½ tsp ground cumin, ½ tsp paprika, ¼ tsp each of onion powder, garlic powder, dried oregano & crushed chilli flakes, 1 tsp each of sea salt & black pepper

Method:

Put everything together in the slow cooker making sure the chicken is covered with the rest of the ingredients. With the lid tightly shut, leave to cook for 4-5 hours on high or 5-6 hours on the low setting. Ensure the chicken is cooked through and tender then shred it a little with 2 forks and serve with a fresh green salad/rice or quesadillas (flour tortilla).

Packed with protein, skinless chicken breasts are a great low fat meat to use in the slow cooker. The citrus lightness of this recipe is perfect

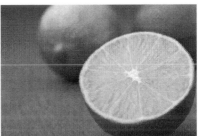

for summer months as well as a welcome taste bud infusion during the colder seasons.

Chicken & Almonds
Serves 4

311 CALORIES PER SERVING

Ingredients:

500g/1lb 2oz skinless chicken breasts, cut into chunks
1 tbsp ground almonds
½ tsp paprika
2 red (bell) peppers, sliced
1 onion, chopped
2 cloves garlic, crushed
1 tbsp white wine vinegar
2 tbsp chopped flat leaf parsley
1 400g/14oz chopped tomatoes

300g/11oz tinned haricot beans, drained
½ tsp dried chilli flakes
100g/3½oz frozen peas
Low cal cooking spray
Salt & pepper to taste

Method:

Brown the chicken pieces in a little low cal spray. Add all the ingredients, except the parsley, into the slow cooker. Season, cover and leave to cook on high for 3-4 hours or low for 5-6 hours. Sprinkle with chopped parsley and serve with rice and/or crusty bread.

This Spanish inspired dish is great as a main meal but can also be served as a delicious ciabatta topping.

BBQ Chicken
Serves 4

Ingredients:

450g/1lb skinless chicken breasts
3 tbsp tomato puree/paste or ketchup
1 tsp each, smoked paprika & garlic powder
60ml/ ¼ cup chicken stock/broth

½ tsp ground cumin & ground coriander/cilantro
1 tbsp brown sugar
3 tbsp Worcestershire sauce
½ tsp salt

Method:

Put all the ingredients into the slow cooker. Mix well, cover and leave to cook on low for 4-5 hours or until the chicken is cooked through and tender. Shred the chicken breasts with 2 forks and mix back into the sauce at the bottom of the slow cooker.

If the sauce needs to be thickened, continue to cook on high for up to 45 mins with the lid off. Alternatively if it's too sticky, add a little water to loosen up. Serve with salad or in sandwich rolls with mayonnaise and BBQ sauce.

When the chicken is shredded and mixed back into the sauce, you should be left with a moist versatile mixture which is effectively the poultry version of the BBQ classic 'pulled pork'.

Lovely Lemony Garlicky Chicken

Serves 4

Ingredients:

500g/1lb 2oz skinless chicken breasts
3 garlic cloves, crushed
2 lemons, sliced
1 onion, chopped
1 tsp runny honey

1 tsp cornstarch dissolved in a little water to make a paste
500ml/2 cups chicken stock/broth
Salt & pepper to taste
Bunch fresh Basil

Method:

Combine all the ingredients in the slow cooker and leave to cook on low for 5-6 hours or on high for 3-4 hours with the lid tightly shut. Ensure the chicken is cooked through and tender. Serve with steamed vegetables and rice to soak up the juices.

This is a really simple dish which really benefits from using fresh lemons and fresh basil ideally.

Luscious Italian Chicken

2 3 5 CALORIES PER SERVING

Serves 4

Ingredients:

500g/1lb 2oz skinless chicken breasts
2 400g/14oz tins low fat condensed chicken or mushroom soup
100g/3 ½ oz mushrooms, sliced
1 onion, chopped
Salt & pepper to taste
1 garlic clove, crushed
2 tbsp fat free cream cheese
Dried rub mix of:
1 teaspoon each oregano, rosemary & thyme

Method:

Rub the chicken breasts with the dried herb mix and combine all the ingredients into the slow cooker. Cook on low for 5-6 hours or on high for 3-4 hours with the lid tightly shut. Ensure the chicken is cooked through and tender; serve with vegetables, spaghetti, rice or noodles.

With a lovely creamy consistency, this Italian inspired dish makes the most of that wonderful 'cheat' ingredient - condensed soup!

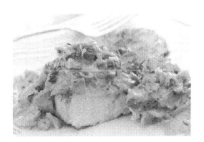

Peanut Butter Chicken

Serves 4

Ingredients:

500g/1lb 2oz skinless chicken breast, diced
1 red (bell) pepper, sliced
1 onion, chopped
4 tbsp low fat peanut butter
2 tbsp lime juice
120ml/ ½ cup chicken stock/ broth
1 tbsp soy sauce
1 tsp each ground cumin & coriander/cilantro
½ tsp paprika
Salt & pepper to taste
Low cal cooking spray

Method:

In a frying pan quickly brown the chicken in a little low cal spray. Add all the ingredients to the slow cooker, season, cover and leave to cook on low for 4-5 hours or high for 3-4 hours. Make sure the chicken is cooked through and serve with noodles & beansprouts.

Peanut butter chicken is delicious. You can really 'lift' the dish by serving with fresh lime wedges.

Mustard Tarragon Chicken

Serves 4

Ingredients:

500g/1lb 2oz skinless chicken breasts
2 tbsp fresh chopped tarragon
1 tsp mild mustard, or more to taste
400g/14oz new potatoes
500ml/2 cups chicken stock/broth

200g/7oz broad beans
200g/7oz tenderstem broccoli
Low cal cooking spray
Salt & pepper to taste
3 tbsp low fat crème fraiche

Method:

Quickly brown the chicken breast in a little low cal spray and thinly slice the potatoes with their skins on. Place all the ingredients, except the crème fraiche, in the slow cooker and season well. Cover and leave to cook on high for 2-3 hours or until the chicken is tender and cooked through. Remove the chicken from the slow cooker, stir through the crème fraiche and pour the vegetable sauce over the chicken.

If you prefer your veg to have some crunch to it, hold off adding to the slow cooker until about 30-45 mins before the end of cooking time.

Simple Chicken Curry

Serves 4

223 CALORIES PER SERVING

Ingredients:

500g/1lb 2oz skinless chicken breasts
1 onion, chopped
1 tbsp tomato puree/paste
3 cloves garlic, crushed
1 tsp low fat butter spread
1 tbsp fresh grated ginger (or use 1 tsp of ginger powder)
1 tsp garam masala
1 tsp ground cumin
1 tsp turmeric
½ tsp chilli powder
250ml/1 cup low fat Greek yoghurt
375ml/1 ½ cups passata/sieved tomatoes
Salt & pepper to taste

Method:

Combine all the ingredients, except the yoghurt, into the slow cooker. Cook on low for 5-6 hours or on high for 3-4 hours with the lid tightly shut. Ensure the chicken is cooked through and tender, turn off the heat and stir in the yoghurt.

Serve with green beans and naan bread.

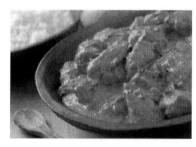

The mix of spices suggested in the recipe is preferable but it is fine to substitute with curry powder if you are in a rush or struggling with store cupboard ingredients.

Chipotle Chicken
Serves 4

198
CALORIES
PER SERVING

Ingredients:

500g/1lb 2oz skinless chicken breasts
1 onion, finely chopped
1 red onion, sliced
3 garlic cloves, crushed
½ tsp brown sugar
2 tsp chipotle paste

1 400g/14oz tin chopped tomatoes
2 tbsp fresh chopped flat leaf parsley
2 tsp sunflower oil
Salt & pepper to taste

Method:

Gently sauté the onion and garlic in the sunflower oil. Remove and quickly brown the chicken breasts in the same pan. Add all the ingredients, except the red onion and parsley, into the slow cooker. Season, cover and leave to cook on high for 2-3 hours or low for 4-5 hours until the meat is tender and cooked through. Shred the chicken with two forks, mix well and serve with the parsley and raw red onion slices on top. Also good with a dollop of fat free Greek yoghurt on the side.

Chipotle paste is essentially smokey chilli paste from the Mexican Chipotle chilli. If you have difficulty sourcing, just substitute for regular chillies and a little smoked paprika.

Chicken & Mustard Leeks
Serves 4

Ingredients:

500g/1lb 2oz skinless chicken breasts
1 tbsp plain flour
100g/3 ½oz lean back bacon
2 leeks, chopped
2 tbsp Dijon mustard
1 tsp mustard powder
250ml/1 cup chicken stock/broth

200g/7oz potatoes, cut into slices
1 bay leaf
300g/11oz spinach
Low cal cooking spray
Salt & pepper to taste

Method:

Season the chicken and coat well in the flour. Add a little low cal spray to a frying pan and quickly brown the breasts. Add all the ingredients to the slow cooker, cover, stir well and leave to cook on high for 2-3 hours or low for 4-5 hours. Remove the chicken from the slow cooker, slice into diagonal strips and ladle the spinach & potato mixture over the top – along with as much of the sauce as you prefer. If you need more liquid during cooking add a little more stock.

The mustard in this recipe should be adjusted to your own taste. You can also use whole grain mustard if you prefer.

Chicken, Garlic & Wine
Serves 4

Ingredients:

500g/1lb 2oz skinless chicken breasts
1 lemon, sliced
2 onions, chopped
6 garlic cloves, sliced

120ml/ ½ cup dry white wine
120ml/ ½ cup chicken stock/ broth
150g/5oz French beans
Salt & pepper to taste

Method:

Season the chicken. Add a little low cal spray to a frying pan and quickly brown the breasts. Add all the ingredients to the slow cooker. Cover, stir well and leave to cook on high for 2-3 hours or low for 4-5 hours. Serve with crusty bread to mop up the delicious lemon juices. If you need more liquid during cooking add a little more stock.

If you prefer your beans crunchy you can hold off adding them until about 20 minutes before the end of cooking.

Chicken & Apricots
Serves 4

225 CALORIES PER SERVING

Ingredients:

500g/1lb 2oz skinless chicken breasts
1 tbsp plain flour
2 garlic cloves, crushed
1 tbsp freshly grated ginger
1 tsp each ground cumin & coriander/cilantro
½ tsp ground cinnamon

1 tsp runny honey
1 tbsp lemon juice
1 400g/14oz tin apricots (in juice)
½ cup/120ml chicken stock/broth
Salt & pepper to taste

Method:

Mix the flour, cinnamon, cumin & coriander together and combine with the chicken breasts.

Add all the other ingredients, except the apricots, but including the apricot juice to the slow cooker. Stir well, cover and leave to cook on high for 2-3 hours or low for 4-5 hours. Add the apricots to the mixture, leave to warm through and serve with steamed greens.

Adding the apricots towards the end of the cooking time prevents them becoming a pulp and retains their form.

Skinny
SLOW COOKER
BEEF DISHES

Italian Meatballs
Serves 5

323
CALORIES
PER SERVING

Ingredients:

650g/1lb 7oz lean minced/
ground beef
1 slice bread, whizzed into
bread crumbs
½ onion finely chopped
Handful fresh parsley chopped
1 large free range egg
1 clove garlic crushed

½ tsp salt
2 400g/14 oz tins chopped
tomatoes
2 tbsp tomato puree/paste
250ml/1 cup beef stock/broth
1 tsp each dried basil, oregano
& thyme

Method:

Combine together the beef, breadcrumbs, egg, onion, garlic and
half the salt. (You can do it with your hands or for super-speed put
it all into a food mixer).

Once the ingredients are properly mixed together, use your hands
to shape into about 20-24 meat balls. Add all the ingredients to
the slow cooker and combine well. Cover and leave to cook on low
for 5-6 hours or 3-4 hours on high. Ensure the beef is well cooked
and serve with spaghetti, parmesan and a green salad.

*Meatballs are easy to make
and never a disappointment
to eat. The simple sauce
accompanying the meat
here is lovely as it is, but
a dash of Worcestershire
sauce or a tsp of marmite
will give it additional depth.*

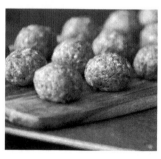

Budapest's Best Beef Goulash

228 CALORIES PER SERVING

Serves 6

Ingredients:

900g/2 lbs lean stewing beef cut into chunks (trim off any fat)
1 red (bell) pepper sliced
3 cloves garlic, crushed
250ml/1 cup beef stock/broth or water
250ml/1 cup red wine

1 400g/14oz tin chopped tomatoes
1 tbsp tomato puree/paste
1 tsp paprika
1 ½ tbsp plain/all purpose flour
1 onion, chopped
Low cal cooking oil
Salt & pepper to taste

Method:

Season the beef and quickly brown in a smoking hot pan with a little low cal spray. Remove from the pan and dust with flour (the easiest way is to put the beef and flour into a plastic bag and give it a good shake). Add all the ingredients to the slow cooker and combine well. Leave to cook on low with the lid tightly shut for 5-6 hours or until the beef is tender and cooked through. If you want to thicken up a little, leave to cook for a further 45 mins with the lid off.

Lovely with a salad & some crusty bread or serve with sour cream and tagliatelle pasta.

Goulash is a European dish which suits the slow cooker beautifully. After hours of gentle cooking this 'tougher' meat becomes a tender cut which just melts in the mouth.

31

Ginger Beef
Serves 6

Ingredients:

675g/1½lb silverside beef/
round steak, cubed
2 garlic cloves, crushed
370ml/1½ cups beef stock/
broth
1 red (bell) pepper, sliced
4 carrots, sliced

1 onion, chopped
2 tbsp soy sauce
1 tbsp freshly grated ginger
1 tbsp corn flour mixed with 3
tbsp water
100g/3½oz frozen peas
Salt & pepper to taste

Method:

Add all the ingredients, except the peas, to the slow cooker.
Season well, cover and leave to cook on low for 5-6 hours or high
for 3-4 hours. An hour before the end of cooking, add the peas
and continue to cook until both the beef and peas are tender.

*Ginger and beef are a great combination and often
used in Chinese cookery. Use low salt soy sauce if you
want to be extra healthy.*

Chilli Con Carne
Serves 4

440
CALORIES
PER SERVING

Ingredients:

550g/1 ¼ lb lean mince/ ground beef
1 400g/14oz tin chopped tomatoes
1 400g/14oz tin kidney beans, drained
1 large onion, chopped
250ml/1 cup beef stock/broth

250ml/1 cup tomato passata/ sieved tomatoes
1 tsp each of brown sugar, oregano, cumin, chilli powder, paprika & garlic powder
½ tsp salt
Low cal cooking spray

Method:

Brown the mince and onions in a frying pan. Add all the ingredients into the slow cooker and combine well. Leave to cook on low for 5-6 hours or high for 3-4 hours with the lid tightly closed. Once the meat is fully cooked through, serve with rice or tortilla chips and a dollop of low fat yoghurt or crème fraiche.

The Spanish name simply means 'chilli with meat' and this dish has been a Tex-Mex classic since before the days of the American frontier settlers. Slow cooking the mince beef really allows the flavour to develop.

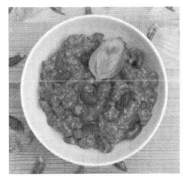

Enchilada El Salvador

Serves 4

Ingredients:

450g/1lb lean minced/ground beef
1 onion, chopped
1 green (bell) pepper, chopped
1 400g/14oz tin black beans, drained
2 400g/14oz tins chopped tomatoes
250ml/1 cup beef stock or boiling water
½ tsp chilli powder

4 tsp taco seasoning
Or make your own:
2 tsp mild chilli powder, 1 ½ tsp ground cumin, ½ tsp paprika, ¼ tsp each of onion powder, garlic powder, dried oregano & crushed chilli flakes, 1 tsp each of sea salt & black pepper

Method:

Add all the ingredients to the slow cooker and combine well. Leave to cook on low with the lid tightly on for 5-6 hours or 3-4 hours on high, until the beef is tender and cooked through. If you want to thicken it up a little leave, to cook for a further 45 mins with the lid off.

Serve with flour tortillas, shredded salad, grated cheese and sour cream (or Greek yoghurt).

Inspired by the flavours of Tex Mex this dish is great fun to eat as a family with everyone helping themselves across the table making their very own perfect enchilada!

Best Beef Brisket
Serves 10

300 CALORIES PER SERVING

Ingredients:

2 ¼ kg/5 lbs beef brisket trimmed of fat
4 large onions, sliced into rounds
500ml/2 cups beef stock/broth or red wine

4 bay leaves
3 garlic cloves, peeled
Salt & pepper to taste

Method:

Season the brisket generously with salt and pepper and brown quickly in a smoking hot dry pan. Lay the onion slices on the bottom of the slow cooker and add the beef along with the rest of the ingredients. Leave to cook with the lid tightly on for 7-9 hours on low. It's best to turn over half way through cooking but don't worry too much if you can't do that. Ensure the beef is super-tender and cooked through. Leave to rest for 20 minutes before slicing.

Brisket is another beef cut which really benefits from the slow cooker as it tenderizes slowly and evenly in its own juices without drying it out.

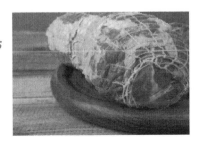

Slow Scottish Stovies
Serves 4

333 CALORIES PER SERVING

Ingredients:

175g/6oz potatoes, diced
2 large onions, chopped
250ml/1 cup vegetable stock/broth

450g/1lb left over roast beef
(or other cooked red meat)
Salt & pepper to taste

Method:

Combine all the ingredients together in the slow cooker and cook on low for 5-6 hours or high for 3-4 hours with the lid tightly shut. The liquid should all be gone by the end of the cooking time, if it hasn't, remove the lid and leave to cook for a little longer. Stir through and serve in bowls with British brown sauce if you have it!

This is a great recipe to use up any cooked leftover red meat you might have. Traditionally it's served with plain Scottish oatcakes and it's super-simple to make. You can also used cubed corned beef in this recipe.

Ragu A La Bolognese
Serves 4

3 4 4
CALORIES
PER SERVING

Ingredients:

500g/1lb 2oz lean minced/ ground beef
1 400g/14oz tin chopped tomatoes
250ml/1 cup passata/sieved tomatoes
1 tsp each dried oregano & thyme

1 stick celery chopped
2 bay leaves
1 tbsp tomato puree/paste
3 garlic cloves, crushed
2 onions, chopped
Salt and pepper to taste
Low cal cooking spray

Method:

Quickly brown the meat in a frying pan with a little low cal spray. Combine all the ingredients in the slow cooker and close the lid tightly. Leave to cook on low for 5-6 hours or high for 3-4 hours. Make sure the meat is cooked through and serve with rigatoni, penne or spaghetti.

Nothing can be simpler or more satisfying than spaghetti bolognese. You can add mushrooms and peppers to the recipe if you like, plus a dash or two of Worcestershire sauce gives extra depth.

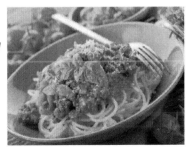

Peppers & Steak
Serves 4

Ingredients:

450g/1lb braising steak/beef chuck
120ml/ ½ cup soy sauce
2 tsp ground black pepper
3 cloves garlic, crushed

3 red or green (bell) peppers, sliced
2 onions, chopped
1 tbsp corn flour
250ml/1 cup water

Method:

Slice the steak and vegetables then add everything to the slow cooker, except the water and corn flour. Season, cover and leave to cook on low for 3-5 hours or until the meat is tender and cooked through. (Add a little water during cooking if the meat becomes too dry). Mix together the corn flour and water into a paste, add to the slow cooker and cook for another 20-30 mins with the lid off or until the sauce is nice and thick.

By slow cooking for a few hours the braising steak should be transformed into a tender cut which can be served on rice or as the heart of a lovely warm salad.

Almonds, Beef & Olives

Serves 4

392 CALORIES PER SERVING

Ingredients:

600g/1lb 5oz lean stewing
steak/chuck steak, cubed
250ml/1 cup beef stock/broth
60ml/¼ cup red wine
1 tsp each smoked paprika,
dried basil & rosemary

1 tbsp plain/all purpose flour
200g/7oz pitted olives
25g/1oz chopped almonds
Salt & pepper to taste

Method:

Season the beef and coat well in the plain flour. Add all the
ingredients, except the olives, to the slow cooker and leave to
cook on low for 4-6 hours or until the beef is tender. Add a little
more stock or wine during cooking if needed and adjust the
seasoning. 20 minutes before the end of cooking add the olives,
warm through and serve.

*This dish is delicious served with creamed spinach
and/or honeyed carrots. Feel free to use a different
mix of dried herbs to suit your taste. You can also
add a tablespoon of tomato puree during cooking to
thicken if you prefer.*

Skinny
SLOW COOKER
PORK DISHES

Perfect Pulled Pork
Serves 6

Ingredients:

900g/2lb pork butt (shoulder)
1 onion, chopped
250ml/1 cup BBQ sauce or
ketchup
250ml/1 cup beef stock/broth
or boiling water
1 packet BBQ dry rub

Or make your own...
1 tbsp each of garlic powder,
brown sugar, onion powder,
celery salt, paprika + 1 tsp each
mild chilli powder & cumin

Method:

Combine all the spices together and cover the pork in the dry
spice rub. Add the stock, onion & BBQ sauce and then place
the pork on top. Leave to cook on high for 6-8 hours with the
lid tightly closed. Ideally you should turn the pork over half way
through cooking, but if you can't do that don't worry. Once the
pork is tender remove it from the slow cooker. Leave to rest for
as long as you can resist and then use your hands or 2 forks to
pull the pork apart. Once it's all shredded, place in a bowl and
remove the cooking liquid from the slow cooker. Pour the liquid
onto the pork to make beautiful juicy meat. Enjoy with just about
everything, whether it's a light salad or sandwich rolls with BBQ
sauce and salad.

*Pulled pork is an absolute
classic. It's a chance to use
just about everything in
your spice rack to create a
'killer' dry rub and it always
packs an irresistible punchy
and more-ish taste.*

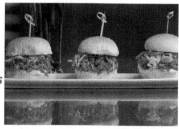

Sausage & Spinach With Gnocchi

Serves 4

309 CALORIES PER SERVING

Ingredients:

6 pork or beef sausages (skins removed)
250ml/1 cup passata/sieved tomatoes
1 tsp dried rosemary
2 tbsp tomato puree/paste
½ tsp brown sugar

1 splash red wine vinegar
½ tsp salt
1 400g/14oz tin chopped tomatoes
100g/ 3½ oz fresh spinach
500g/1lb 2oz gnocchi

Method:

Brown the sausage meat in a frying pan and break up well. Add all the ingredients, except the gnocchi and spinach, to the slow cooker and combine. Close the lid tightly and leave to cook on high for 3-4 hours. When the meat is well cooked, stir in the fresh spinach, gnocchi and leave to cook for a further 10-20 mins or until the gnocchi is tender.

This lovely recipe uses sausage meat to create a thick, luxurious sauce which is just perfect with freshly cooked gnocchi. You can also add some crushed chilli if you prefer a 'kick' of heat.

Cowboy Casserole
Serves 4

414 CALORIES PER SERVING

Ingredients:

8 lean pork sausages
2 400g/14oz tins mixed beans, drained
2 400g/14oz tins chopped tomatoes
1 onion, chopped
2 carrots, chopped

1 tbsp tomato puree/paste or ketchup
1 tsp brown sugar
1 tsp Dijon/mild mustard
Low cal cooking spray

Method:

Brown the sausages in the pan with the onions. Combine all the ingredients in the slow cooker and leave to cook for 3-4 hours on high or low for 5-6 hours with the lid tightly shut. Check the sausages are properly cooked through and, if you want to thicken the sauce up, leave the lid off while you cook on high for up to 45 mins extra.

Serve on its own with crusty bread or with mashed potato and green veg.

Loved by kids and adults alike, this is a real cowboy's supper-time meal which always goes down a treat. It takes just minutes to put together and is a great way to get some vegetables into the kids.

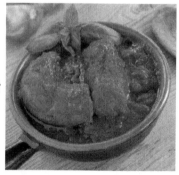

Aromatic Kicking Pork Ribs

Serves 5

Ingredients:

1kg/2 ¼ lbs pork ribs
1 tsp each garlic powder, chilli, cumin & basil
½ tsp salt
2 400g/14oz tins chopped tomatoes

1 tbsp ketchup
1 green chilli, chopped or pinch crushed chilli flakes to taste

Method:

Rub the dry spices onto the ribs. Add all the ingredients to the slow cooker and leave to cook with the lid tightly on for 5-6 hours on low. Ensure the ribs are super tender and serve with rice and beans.

There are a number of different types of rib available depending on the cut from which they are taken. Choose whichever is cheapest or whichever you prefer. All will work well with this recipe.

Sweet & Sour Pineapple Pork

Serves 6

238 CALORIES PER SERVING

Ingredients:

900g/2lb lean cubed pork
1 tbsp plain/all purpose flour
1 400g/14oz tin pineapple chunks (reserve the juice)
1 onion, chopped
1 green (bell) pepper, chopped
2 carrots, cut into batons

1 tbsp brown sugar
½ tsp salt
2 tbsp lime juice
1 tbsp light soy sauce
120ml/½ cup boiling water
Low cal cooking spray

Method:

Brown the pork in a frying pan with a little low cal spray. Remove from the pan and dust with the flour. Put all the other ingredients, except the pineapple chunks, into the slow cooker (include the pineapple juice). Combine everything and leave to cook on low for 4-5 hours with the lid tightly closed. Check the pork is tender and then add the pineapple chunks. Leave for a further 30 min and serve with boiled rice.

Sweet and sour is one of the most loved Chinese meals in the world. This is not supposed to be an authentic copy - just take it as a super simple replica which should satisfy your eastern cravings.

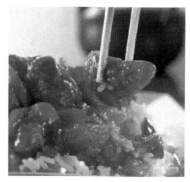

Cumin Pork & Kidney Beans

366 CALORIES PER SERVING

Serves 6

Ingredients:

1 400g/14oz tin kidney beans, drained
300g/11oz lean boneless pork shoulder, cubed
1 onion, chopped
4 garlic cloves, crushed

1 tsp sunflower oil
1 tsp ground cumin
½ tsp turmeric
250ml/1 cup vegetable stock/broth
Salt & pepper to taste

Method:

Quickly brown the cubed pork in a frying pan with the sunflower oil. Add all the ingredients to the slow cooker and season well. Cover and leave to cook on high for 3-4 hours or low for 5-6 hours, or until the pork is tender and cooked through. If you want to thicken the sauce a little, leave the lid off and cook for an additional 45 mins, or until you have the consistency you prefer.

This pork dish is great served with rice and sour cream. You could also garnish with some fresh finely chopped chillies.

Lentils, Sausages & Peas

Serves 4

390 CALORIES PER SERVING

Ingredients:

50g/2oz red lentils
½ tsp each crushed chilli flakes, ground cumin & coriander/cilantro
1 onion, sliced
450g/1lb lean pork sausages
120ml/½ cup beef stock/broth

150g/5oz frozen peas
1 tbsp Dijon mustard
2 tbsp freshly chopped flat leaf parsley
Low cal cooking spray
Salt & pepper to taste

Method:

Add a little low cal spray to a frying pan and quickly brown the sausages. Add all the ingredients to the slow cooker, stir well, cover and leave to cook on high for 2-3 hours or low for 4-5 hours. If you need more liquid during cooking add a little more stock. Ensure the lentils are tender and the sausages cooked through. Serve with boiled potatoes and spinach.

You can serve the sausages whole or alternatively remove after cooking, slice in diagonals, return to the slow cooker and stir through before serving.

Skinny
SLOW COOKER
LAMB DISHES

Lamb Pilau Pazar
Serves 4

Ingredients:

500g/1lb 2oz lean lamb cut into bite sized chunks (any lean cut will work for this recipe)
1 large onion, chopped
1 carrot, chopped
1 stick celery, chopped
1 400g/14oz tin chopped tomatoes
1 tsp dried crushed chilli flakes
150g/5 oz brown rice
500ml/2 cups vegetable stock/broth
1 cinnamon stick or ½ tsp ground cinnamon
25g/1oz dried apricots or raisins
Salt & pepper to taste
Low cal cooking spray

Method:

Gently sauté the onion in a little low cal spray, remove from the pan and then brown off the lamb for a couple of minutes on a high heat. Combine all the ingredients together in the slow cooker, except the rice. Cover and cook on low for 4-6 hours, add the rice and cook for 30 mins or until the rice and lamb are both tender and cooked through.

If any additional liquid remains, cook on a high heat with the lid off for a further 45 minutes or until the liquid is absorbed into the rice.

If you want to add garnish serve with toasted pine nuts, chopped coriander/cilantro or crushed almonds.

Also known as pilaf, Pilau is a rice based dish now common just about everywhere. The version here has a taste of the Turkish to it hence its title Pazar which means 'Sunday' and is also the name of a beautiful coastal village in the Rize province of the country.

Spinach & Lamb Stew

Serves 4

467
CALORIES
PER SERVING

Ingredients:

500g/1lb 2oz lean lamb cut into bite sized chunks (any lean cut will work)
2 cloves garlic, crushed
Zest of 1 lemon
1 onion, chopped
2 400g/14oz tins chopped tomatoes
1 tbsp tomato puree/paste
1 400g/14oz tin chickpeas, drained

400g/14oz fresh spinach, chopped
Dried herb mix of the following:
1 tsp each coriander/cilantro & turmeric
½ tsp each ground cumin, black pepper & oregano
2 tbsp low fat Greek yoghurt
Salt & pepper to taste
Low cal cooking spray

Method:

Gently sauté the onion in a little low cal oil, remove from the pan and then brown the lamb for a couple of minutes on a high heat. Combine all ingredients together (except the yoghurt and spinach) in the slow cooker with the lid tightly shut and cook on low for 4-6 hours or until the lamb is tender and cooked through. 30mins before the end of cooking add the spinach, stir through the yoghurt before serving.

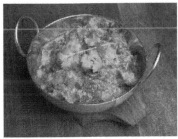

Super rich in iron & calcium, spinach is a super-food which is twinned beautifully in this dish with chickpeas, lemon zest and Greek inspired spices.

Marrakesh Lamb
Serves 4

4 1 5
CALORIES
PER SERVING

Ingredients:

500g/1lb 2oz trimmed lamb cut into cubes (any lean cut will work)
½ tsp black pepper
1 tsp each ground cumin, coriander, ginger, turmeric & paprika
1 tsp cinnamon

2 400g/14oz tins chopped tomatoes
75g/3oz red split lentils
1 lt/4 cups lamb stock/broth or boiling water
2 onions, chopped
1 tsp brown sugar
5 cloves garlic, crushed

Method:

This one couldn't be any easier. No need to brown the meat, so just combine all the ingredients in the slow cooker, cover and leave to cook on low for 4-6 hours. Ensure the lamb is tender and cooked through. If you want to thicken up a little, leave to cook for a further 45 mins with the lid off.

Delicious served with low fat Greek yoghurt, couscous or fragrant rice.

Morocco's capital is world renowned for its tagine cuisine. Slow cookers provide a wonderful alternative to this specialist style of cooking. This recipe is a 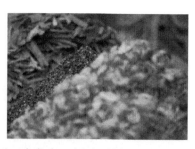 *lovely North African inspired dish which, if its new to you, should piqué your interest in Moroccan cooking.*

Lamb & Saag Spinach

320 CALORIES PER SERVING

Serves 4

Ingredients:

500g/1lb 2oz lean lamb shoulder, cubed
1 tsp each fenugreek & mustard seeds
1 tsp each ground cumin & ginger

2 cloves garlic, crushed
250ml/1 cup beef stock/broth
400g/14oz spinach
120ml/½ cup fat free Greek yoghurt
1 tsp mint sauce (shop bought)

Method:

Other than the yoghurt and mint sauce add all the ingredients to the slow cooker, cover and leave to cook on low for 4-6 hours or until the lamb is tender. Stir the yoghurt and mint sauce through and serve straight away.

Saag means 'leaf' dish in Indian cuisine. You could try out other green leaves as an alternative to spinach if you prefer.

Skinny
SLOW COOKER
SEAFOOD DISHES

Green Thai Fish Curry

Serves 4

Ingredients:

500g/1lb 2oz meaty white fish fillets (go for whatever is on sale) haddock, cod, Pollock or cobbler

3 onions, chopped

1 tsp fresh ginger or ½ tsp ground ginger

3 cloves garlic, crushed

1 red chilli, chopped

50g/2oz watercress

2 tbsp Thai green curry paste

500ml/ 2 cups low fat coconut milk

150g/5oz green beans

Low cal cooking spray

Salt & pepper to taste

Method:

Sauté the onions & green beans with the ginger and garlic over a low heat in a little low cal spray. Season the fish fillets and carefully combine all the ingredients (except the watercress) in the slow cooker. Cook on low for 1 ½ hours with the lid tightly shut. This timing should mean your fish is not overcooked and the green beans have some bite to them. Check the fish is properly cooked through by flaking it a little with a fork and gently add the watercress salad to the mix before serving. Serve with noodles or rice.

If you want to make it a little spicier you could add some more chopped chilli or crushed chilli flakes.

Compared to meat, fish cooks more quickly in the slow cooker and as such fish recipes can be really handy if you haven't got too much cooking time. This recipe is a fantastic and easy Thai curry 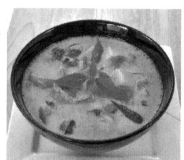 *which is simple to prepare and doesn't take long at all in the slow cooker.*

Sweet & Citrus Salmon

Serves 4

270 CALORIES PER SERVING

Ingredients:

500g/1lb 2oz thick boneless salmon fillets
1 onion, chopped
1 tbsp light soy sauce
Juice of 1 fresh lime or 3 tbsp Lime juice

2 garlic cloves, crushed
1 tsp sugar dissolved into 3 tbsp warm water and brushed onto the fillets
Low cal cooking spray
Salt & pepper to taste

Method:

Chop the onion and sauté for a couple of minutes with the garlic in a little low cal oil. Remove from the pan and carefully combine all the ingredients in the slow cooker. Cook on low for 1½ hours with the lid tightly on. Check the fish is properly cooked by flaking it a little with a fork and serve with salad potatoes and carrots. Alternatively, use in a lovely warm salad served with a little crusty bread.

Salmon can be relatively expensive so you can substitute for tilapia or basa or talk to your fishmonger for recommendations.

Tuna & Noodle Cattia

Serves 4

250 CALORIES PER SERVING

Ingredients:

350g/12oz fresh egg noodles
1 onion, chopped
1 400g/14oz tin fat free condensed mushroom soup
2 200g/7oz tins tuna steaks or flakes in water

100g/3 ½ oz frozen peas
1 tsp garlic powder
Salt & pepper to taste
Pinch of crushed chilli flakes

Method:

Quickly cook the pasta or noodles in salted boiling water. Save 3 tbsp of the drained water and then combine all the ingredients and saved water in the slow cooker. Cover and leave to cook on low for 1½ hours.

This is great served with a sliced red onion & tomato salad and a little parmesan.

An absolute classic American slow cooker recipe, Tuna & Noodle casserole is always a winner. This version takes it back to basics using the simplest store cupboard ingredients. The title 'Cattia' pays homage to the ancient Latin roots where the word 'casserole' has its origins.

Coriander & Garlic Prawns

269 CALORIES PER SERVING

Serves 4

Ingredients:

500g/1lb2oz raw king prawns
200g/7oz frozen peas
1 tsp sunflower oil
2 onions, sliced
200g/8oz cherry tomatoes, halved
1 tsp ground ginger

4 garlic cloves, crushed
3 tbsp curry paste
2 tbsp fresh chopped coriander/cilantro
250ml/1 cup passata/sieved tomatoes
Salt & pepper to taste

Method:

Add all the ingredients to the slow cooker, cover and leave to cook on low for 1-2 hours or until the prawns are cooked through and the peas are tender. Sprinkle with chopped coriander and serve with rice.

This is a really simple 'cheat' curry using curry paste. If you want a slightly different taste you could use less passata and add a little coconut milk to the recipe after cooking.

Fish Stew
Serves 4

245
CALORIES
PER SERVING

Ingredients:

450g/1lb white fish fillets, cubed
1 leek, chopped
4 garlic cloves, crushed
1 400g/14oz tin chopped tomatoes
100g/3 ½ oz frozen peas

2 stalk celery, chopped
1 onion chopped
½ tsp fennel seeds
1 tbsp dried basil
1lt/4 cups fish stock/broth
250g/9oz raw prawns
Salt & Pepper to taste

Method:

Mix together all the ingredients, except the fish, peas and prawns in the slow cooker. Season, cover and leave to cook on low for 4-5 hours or high for 2-3 hours. Meanwhile season the fish and prawns. 45 mins before the end of cooking add the fish, prawns and peas. Continue to cook until the seafood is cooked right through and the peas are tender. Serve with noodles as a soup stew.

Feel free to use any type of meaty white fish you like and, if you feel adventurous, you could add some squid, octopus or clams to the stew.

Skinny
SLOW COOKER
VEGETARIAN DISHES

Pomodoro Pasta Sauce

Serves 4

Ingredients:

2 400g/14oz tins chopped tomatoes
6 large fresh tomatoes (vine ripened are best)
250ml/1 cup passata/sieved tomatoes
Handful sliced black olives
Bunch fresh basil chopped (reserve a little some for garnish)
3 garlic cloves, crushed
1 onion, chopped
1 tsp brown sugar
1 tsp extra virgin olive oil
Salt and pepper to taste

Method:

Combine all the ingredients in the slow cooker and cover. Leave to cook on low for 5-6 hours or high for 3-4 hours. Delicious served with angel hair pasta, salad & grated parmesan cheese.

This is a simple tomato based Italian sauce which gets better the longer you leave it. Reheated leftovers often have a greater depth of taste which is worth waiting for.

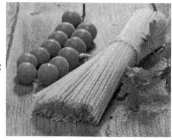

Veggie Turmeric Chickpeas

234 CALORIES PER SERVING

Serves 4

Ingredients:

2 400g/14oz tins chickpeas, drained
2 onions, chopped
1 tbsp tomato puree/paste
2 cloves garlic, crushed
1 tsp fresh grated ginger or ½ teaspoon ground ginger
2 tsp garam masala
1 tsp each ground cumin & coriander/cilantro
2 tsp turmeric
½ tsp chilli powder
200g/7oz fresh spinach
3 tbsp lemon juice
250ml/1 cup veg stock/broth
Salt & pepper to taste

Method:

Combine all the ingredients, except the lemon juice and spinach, in the slow cooker. Cook on low for 5-6 hours or on high for 3-4 hours with the lid tightly shut. Add a little more stock during cooking if needed. Ensure the chickpeas are cooked though, stir in the lemon juice and spinach. Serve with rice and naan bread.

Chickpeas have been used in cooking for many hundreds of years. The spinach in this recipe will be crunchy, if you prefer your spinach well cooked, add earlier during cooking.

Tomato & Garlic Mushrooms

Serves 4

180
CALORIES
PER SERVING

Ingredients:

1 tbsp olive oil
450g/1lb chestnut mushrooms
5 cloves garlic, crushed
1 stick celery
1 400g/14oz tin chopped tomatoes

1 tbsp tomato puree/paste
3 tbsp fresh chopped flat leaf parsley
½ tsp crushed chilli flakes
1 onion, chopped

Method:

Add all the ingredients to the slow cooker, except the parsley. Season, cover and leave to cook on high for 3-4 hours or low for 5-6 hours or until the mushrooms are tender and the flavours have thoroughly blended.

This is great served with spaghetti & salad for a delicious Italian meal, or on bruschetta as a snack.

Fennel Risotto
Serves 3

Ingredients:

1 fennel bulb, diced
250g/9oz risotto rice
1 carrot, chopped
1 onion, chopped
25g/1oz grated parmesan cheese
50g/2oz black olives, finely chopped

3 garlic cloves, crushed
1lt/4 cups vegetable stock/ broth
125g/4oz frozen peas
50g/2oz rocket
15g/ ½ oz butter
Salt & pepper to taste

Method:

Preheat the slow cooker and place the butter in the bottom. When it is melted, add the risotto rice and stir well until every grain is finely coated. Add the rest of the ingredients, except the cheese and rocket, to the slow cooker and season well. Cover and leave to cook on high for 2-3 hours. If you need to add more liquid during cooking go ahead by adding just a little each time. After cooking, all the liquid should be absorbed and the rice should be tender. If it isn't, leave to cook for a little longer with the lid off. Serve sprinkled with parmesan cheese and the rocket piled on top.

Risotto usually needs a lot of stirring during cooking. This slow cooker alternative is a great labour saver with virtually no stirring required.

Wild Mushroom Stroganoff

101
CALORIES
PER SERVING

Serves 4

Ingredients:

500g/1lb 2oz wild mixed
mushrooms sliced
2 onions, chopped
4 garlic cloves, crushed
2 tsp smoked paprika
250ml/1 cup vegetable stock/
broth

1 400g/14oz tin low fat
condensed mushroom soup
Bunch flat chopped leaf parsley
(reserve a little for garnish)

Method:

Add all the ingredients into the slow cooker. Close the lid tightly
and leave to cook on high for 2-3 hours or low for 4-5 hours.
Ensure the mushrooms are tender and serve with pasta or rice
and a spoon of fat free Greek yoghurt.

*The more exciting the
mushrooms the better
this dish is going to
taste. Use whatever you
can get your hands on
but a combination of
portobello, shitake,*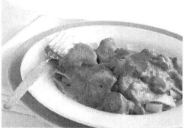
*morel, oyster and enoki would be fantastic. However
don't be put off if you can only get regular varieties -
it will still taste good!*

Bean, Potato & Cheese Stew

Serves 4

434 CALORIES PER SERVING

Ingredients:

1 400g/14oz tin sweetcorn
2 400g/14oz tins mixed beans, drained
1 red (bell) pepper, chopped
1 onion, chopped
500ml/2 cups passata/sieved tomatoes
1 tsp each cumin & coriander/cilantro

Salt & pepper to taste
125g/4oz grated low fat cheese
125g/4oz potatoes, diced & peeled
½ tsp cayenne pepper
Juice of one lemon or 2tbsp lemon juice

Method:

Add all the ingredients to the slow cooker, except the cheese. Combine well and sprinkle the cheese onto the top. Cook on low for 5-6 hours or on high for 3-4 hours with the lid tightly shut. Make sure the potatoes are tender and serve with sour cream and flat bread. If you find the stew is a little dry during cooking, add some water to loosen.

This vegetarian meal is a lovely Mexican inspired dish which is so hearty, you won't miss the meat at all. Feel free to spice it up with extra cayenne pepper if you like and serve with an onion & tomato or green salad.

Lentil Dhal
Serves 4

160 CALORIES PER SERVING

Ingredients:

400g/14oz split red lentils
1 onion, chopped
1 garlic clove, crushed
1 tsp each ground coriander/
cilantro, turmeric & cumin
½ each tsp ground ginger,
paprika & mustard seeds

500ml/2 cups vegetable stock/
broth
2 tbsp freshly chopped
coriander/cilantro
25g/1oz butter
Salt & pepper to taste

Method:

Add all the ingredients to the slow cooker, cover and leave to cook on low for 4-6 hours or until the lentils are tender and the liquid absorbed. Add a little more stock or water during cooking if needed. If there is too much liquid, take the lid off and leave to cook on high for approx 40 mins. Sprinkle the chopped coriander over the top and serve.

Dhal is a one of the most common dishes in Asia. It is eaten by some families at almost every single meal time. This simple version is great served with Indian chapatti bread.

Butter Bean & Almond Stew

Serves 4

206 CALORIES PER SERVING

Ingredients:

1 onion, sliced into rounds
2 garlic cloves, crushed
300g/11oz new potatoes, sliced
1 tsp mustard seeds
2 tbsp tomato puree/paste
½ tsp ground cinnamon
1 celery stick, chopped
450g/1lb cauliflower florets
50g/2oz sultanas

200g/7oz tinned butter beans, drained
50g/2oz chopped almonds
1 400g/14oz tin chopped tomatoes
250ml/1 cup vegetable stock/broth
Salt & pepper to taste

Method:

Add all the ingredients to the slow cooker, cover, stir well and leave to cook on high for 2-3 hours or low for 4-5 hours or until the vegetables are tender.

If you want the stew a little thicker, take the lid off and continue to cook on high for 45mins or until the consistency is to your liking.

Skinny
SLOW COOKER
SOUPS

Hock Ham & Split Pea Soup

Serves 4

Ingredients:

2 ham knuckles (get them smoked if you can)
3 carrots, chopped
2 celery stalks, chopped
1 onion chopped

3 garlic cloves, crushed
500g/1lb 2oz green split peas (yellow or green are fine)
1 ½ lt/6 cups chicken stock/ broth

Method:

Combine all the ingredients into the slow cooker and cook on low for 5-6 hours or high for 3-4 hours with the lid tightly shut. When the soup is cooked, take out the hocks and strip the meat - if they are fully cooked the meat should fall away easily. Discard any fat and stir the shredded ham back into the soup. If you want to alter the texture you can thicken it up by mashing the split peas a little before putting the ham back in.

Ham hocks are a bargain ingredient that can give a real depth to a dish. You could substitute ham hocks for a meaty ham bone if you had one left after a family gathering.

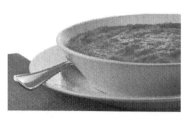

Super Simple Chicken Taco Soup

Serves 6

Ingredients:

125g/4oz skinless chicken breast
1 400g/14oz tin sweetcorn
1 400g/14oz tin black beans, drained
1 400g/14oz tin kidney bean, drained
1 400g/14oz tin chopped tomatoes
2 cloves garlic, crushed
1 ¼lt/5 cups chicken stock/broth

1 red chilli, chopped
4 tsp taco seasoning
Or make your own
1 tbsp chilli powder, 1 ½ tsp ground cumin, ½ tsp paprika, ¼ tsp each of onion powder, garlic powder, dried oregano & crushed chilli flakes, 1 tsp each of sea salt & black pepper

Method:

Season the chicken breast and place at the bottom of the slow cooker. Add all the other ingredients and leave to cook for 2 hours on high or 3 hours on low with the lid tightly shut. Ensure the chicken is cooked through and tender then shred it a little with 2 forks through the soup.

If you want to thicken the soup up after cooking, take the lid off and cook on high for a further 45 minutes or until you get the consistency you want.

Serve with tortilla chips, crusty bread or over rice depending on how much of a meal you want to make of it.

No one knows when Taco turned into soup, but whenever it was it has become a firm favourite which is worth celebrating in the slow cooker.

Squash, Basil & Tomato Soup

Serves 4

Ingredients:

400g/14oz butternut squash flesh, cubed
75g/3oz potatoes, peeled & cubed
8 fresh vine tomatoes, chopped
½ tsp sugar
2 tbsp freshly chopped basil leaves

4 tbsp tomato puree/paste
1lt/4 cups vegetable stock/broth
60ml/¼ cup single cream
Salt & pepper to taste

Method:

Place all the ingredients, except the cream, in the slow cooker. Season, cover and leave to cook on low for 3-4 hours or until the vegetables are tender. After cooking blend the soup to a smooth consistency and serve with a swirl of fresh cream.

Butternut squash is a perfect slow cooker ingredient. Its creamy, firm texture holds well during cooking and forms a robust base to this tasty soup.

Spanish Sausage Soup

Serves 4

Ingredients:

75g/3oz potatoes, cubed
450g/1lb cauliflower florets, finely chopped
1 tbsp olive oil
750ml/3 cups vegetable stock/ broth
250ml/1 cup semi skimmed milk
2 tbsp freshly chopped flat leaf parsley
1 tsp smoked paprika
100g/3 ½ oz chorizo sausage, finely chopped
Salt & pepper to taste

Method:

Place all the ingredients, except the parsley, in the slow cooker. Season, cover and leave to cook on low for 3-4 hours or until the vegetables are tender. Adjust the seasoning and serve with the parsley sprinkled on top.

Chorizo sausage is quintessentially Spanish. You can use either the cooked, cured or raw versions of chorizo for this recipe.

St.Patrick's Day Soup
Serves 4

Ingredients:

300g/11oz potatoes chopped
1 onion, chopped
3 leeks, chopped
Salt & pepper to taste

500ml/2 cups skimmed milk
750ml/3 cups vegetable stock/
broth

Method:

Combine all the ingredients together in the slow cooker and leave
to cook on low for 4-5 hours with the lid tightly shut. Make sure
the potatoes are tender, season to taste and then either blend as
a smooth soup or eat it rough, ready and rustic with some crusty
bread.

You can also add a garnish of chopped chives and sour cream or
crème fraiche if you want to add an extra touch.

*It's often said that
everyone is Irish on St.
Patrick's day, here's a
chance to get a real taste
of Ireland every day with
this lovely Irish inspired
potato soup.*

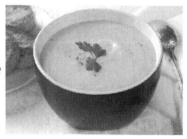

Spicy Carrot Soup
Serves 4

Ingredients:

2 tsp ground cumin
½ tsp crushed chilli flakes
1 tbsp olive oil
750g/1lb 11oz carrots, finely chopped
½ onion, finely chopped

140g/4 ½ oz split red lentils
750ml/3 cups vegetable stock/broth
120ml/ ½ cup milk
60ml/ ¼ cup single cream
Salt & pepper to taste.

Method:

Add all the ingredients to the slow cooker, except the cream and milk. Season, cover and leave to cook on high for approx 3 hours or until the lentils are tender. Add the milk and warm through for a minute or two. Use a food processor or blender to whizz the soup to a smooth consistency and serve with a swirl of single cream in each bowl.

This warming soup can be tweaked to suit your taste - add more or less chilli flakes as you prefer. Plus if you want to reduce the calories a little, swap the olive oil for low cal cooking spray and the regular milk for skimmed.

Flageolet & Savoy Soup

Serves 4

Ingredients:

1 onion, finely chopped
1 carrot, finely chopped
1 whole savoy cabbage, chopped
1 tbsp olive oil
1lt/4 cups vegetable stock/broth

2 tbsp tomato puree/paste
1 tsp each dried oregano & rosemary
Salt & Pepper to taste
1 400g/14oz tin flageolet beans, drained

Method:

Place all the ingredients in the slow cooker. Season, cover and leave to cook on low for 3-4 hours or until the vegetables are tender. Adjust the seasoning and serve.

This soup is best served chunky. If however, you prefer a smoother consistency, reserve a ladle of flageolet beans from the cooked soup, blend the rest of the soup and stir the whole beans back through before serving.

Parsnip & Coconut Milk Soup

Serves 4

238
CALORIES
PER SERVING

Ingredients:

1 onion, chopped
4 parsnips, chopped
4 carrots, chopped
1 tsp each turmeric, cumin,
coriander/cilantro & paprika
120ml/ ½ cup low fat coconut
milk

2 tbsp freshly chopped chives
750ml/3 cups vegetable stock/
broth
Salt & pepper to taste
250ml/1 cup fat free Greek
yoghurt

Method:

Place all the ingredients, except the chives, coconut milk &
yoghurt in the slow cooker. Season, cover and leave to cook on
low for 3-4 hours or until the vegetables are tender. After cooking,
blend the soup to a smooth consistency and serve with a dollop of
yoghurt in the middle and some fresh chives sprinkled on top.

*Adding the coconut milk during lengthy cooking risks
the milk 'splitting', so leave it until the end and warm
through.*

Corn & Potato Chowder

Serves 4

230 CALORIES PER SERVING

Ingredients:

1 onion, chopped
400g/14oz sweetcorn
400g/14oz creamed sweetcorn
2 cloves garlic, crushed
750ml/3 cups chicken or vegetable stock/broth
350g/12oz potatoes, diced

1 tsp low fat 'butter' spread
500ml/2 cups semi skimmed milk
Salt & pepper to taste
Low cal cooking spray

Method:

Gently sauté the onion and garlic in a little low cal spray. Place all the ingredients in the slow cooker and cook on low for 3-4 hours with the lid tightly shut. Ensure the potatoes are tender and mash a little with a fork to create the right consistency. Serve with saltine or cream crackers for an authentic finish.

Although primarily associated with seafood, chowder is a lovely thick soup recipe which works just as well with vegetables alone. You could easily add some 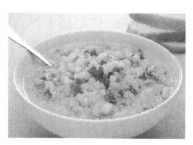 *smoked haddock to this recipe if you wanted to be authentic, but this veggie option is good too.*

Spinach & Haricot Soup

Serves 6

240 CALORIES PER SERVING

Ingredients:

2 lt/8 cups vegetable stock/broth
4 tbsp tomato puree/paste
1 400g/14oz tin haricot beans, rinsed
250g/9oz brown rice

200g/7oz spinach
2 onions, chopped
2 garlic cloves, crushed
1 tsp each dried basil & oregano
Salt & pepper to taste

Method:

Combine all the ingredients, except the spinach, into the slow cooker. Season, cover and leave to cook on low for 5-6 hours or high for 3-4 hours. 20 minutes before the end of cooking, stir through the spinach. Serve with crusty bread.

This hearty soup is great freshened up with a twist of lemon and chopped basil to garnish.

Skinny
SLOW COOKER
BREAKFASTS

Spanish Tortilla
Serves 4

Ingredients:

A dozen eggs, gently fork whisked
One large onion, chopped
150g/5oz potatoes, peeled and cut into thin slices

50g/2 oz cured chorizo Spanish sausage, finely chopped
Salt & pepper to taste
Low cal cooking spray

Method:

Gently sauté the onions and potatoes in a little low cal spray until golden (5-10 mins). Spray the slow cooker with a little more oil and add all the ingredients. Combine well, cover and leave to cook on low overnight for 6-8 hours for a perfect morning feast.

This Spanish omelette makes a fantastic hearty start to the morning. It's also great served cold and cut into slices with a fresh green salad.

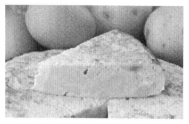

Morning Risotto
Serves 4

271 CALORIES PER SERVING

Ingredients:

175g/6oz risotto rice
4 apples, peeled, cored & sliced
125g/4oz sultanas
1 tsp cinnamon
½ tsp nutmeg

¼ tsp ground cloves
500ml/2 cups water
500ml/2 cups skimmed milk
1 tbsp brown sugar
Knob butter

Method:

Melt the butter in a pan and add the rice. Make sure it's all nicely coated for just a minute or two and then add all the ingredients to the slow cooker. Leave to cook overnight for 6-8 hours with the lid tightly closed. If it feels a little stodgy in the morning loosen it up by stirring a dash of cold milk through.

Another lovely breakfast alternative which uses Italian rice to give the dish its base.

Fruit Granola
Serves 4

Ingredients:

500g/1lb 2oz plain granola
cereal
100g/3 ½ oz oatmeal
1 tsp cinnamon
½ tsp nutmeg

1 tbsp runny honey
4 apples sliced & cored
50g/2oz sultanas
50g/2oz low fat 'butter' spread,
melted

Method:

Add all the ingredients to the slow cooker and combine well.
Cover and leave to cook for 2-3 hours making sure the granola
doesn't burn. Serve with milk if you like.

*This recipe is basically
your favourite granola
cereal combined with
fresh fruit and spices
to fill your kitchen
with a lovely warming,
welcoming aroma.*

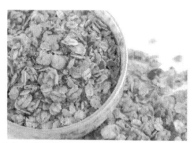

*Also good as a dessert with a little more sugar and a
dob of fresh cream.*

Skinny
SLOW COOKER
SNACKS

Bean, Rosemary & Roasted Garlic Dip

Serves 14

88 CALORIES PER SERVING

Ingredients:

6 garlic cloves chopped
100g/3 ½ oz parmesan cheese grated
1 bunch chopped fresh rosemary
2 tbsp extra virgin olive oil
1 400g/14oz tin borlotti beans, drained

125g/4oz low fat cream cheese
Handful chopped black olives
1 tbsp white wine vinegar
250ml/1 cup water
1 tbsp lemon juice
Salt to taste

Method:

Quickly pulse all the ingredients (except the lemon juice) in a food processor. Empty the blitzed mixture into the slow cooker and leave to cook on low for 1-2 hours. If the mixture is too thick, add a little more water. If it's not thick enough, continue to cook with the lid off until you get the required consistency. After cooking allow to cool, stir in the lemon juice and serve with a selection of raw celery, cucumber and carrot batons.

This is a perfect low cal snack to keep you going between meals.

Nacho Bean & Onion Dip

Serves 12

Ingredients:

2 400g/14oz tins low fat refried beans
1 green chilli, finely chopped
1 onion, chopped
100g/3 ½ oz mozzarella cheese chopped
4 tsp taco seasoning mix
250ml/1 cup water

Or make your own:
2 tsp mild chilli powder, 1 ½ tsp ground cumin, ½ tsp paprika, ¼ tsp each of onion powder, garlic powder, dried oregano & crushed chilli flakes, 1 tsp each of sea salt & black pepper
Salt to taste
1 tbsp lemon juice

Method:

Place all the ingredients, except the lemon juice, into the slow cooker and combine well. Leave to cook on low for 1-2 hours and before serving, stir in the lemon juice. If the mixture is too thick add a little more water. If it's not thick enough, continue to cook with the lid off until you get the required consistency. Serve warm with plain tortilla chips.

Buffallo mozzarella is good in this recipe but regular mozzarella is fine too. Use the full fat versions of both.

Honey Roasted Vegetables

281 CALORIES PER SERVING

Serves 6
Ingredients:

250g/9oz carrots
250g/9oz parsnips
1 tbsp balsamic vinegar
3 tsp runny honey
2 red onions
2 red (bell) peppers
2 tbsp olive oil

1 tsp each ground cumin, paprika, & chilli powder
½ tsp ground cinnamon
200g/7oz tinned chopped tomatoes
Salt & pepper to taste

Method:

Peel and cut the carrots, parsnips, peppers and onions into chunks. Combine all the ingredients well in the slow cooker. Season, cover and leave to cook on low for 3-4 hours or until the vegetables are tender. Add a little water during cooking if needed.

This is a great Moroccan inspired dish which is also nice with some chopped apricots if you like additional sweetness.

Skinny
SLOW COOKER
CURRIES

Bonus Takeaway Curry Section

We hope you enjoy this bonus curry section of 'The Skinny Slow Cooker Recipe Book'. Following a huge response from readers we developed 'The Skinny Indian Takeaway Recipe Book'. Here we have included some of the favourite recipes so you can try takeaway curry cooking yourself.

Indian food has never been more popular, but it's easy to be overwhelmed by the idea of Indian cooking. With the cuisine relying so heavily on spice blends, you can be put off by the vast array on offer before you've even started. Don't be afraid of spices - you'll get to know them quickly and become confident in your cooking in no time. These recipes use just a handful of key spices which you can use time and time again and which, once bought, you can keep in the store cupboard and go back to month after month - saving you money in the long run.

Serving Sizes

Most of the dishes in this section serve 2. You can alter the quantities to serve more if you like, however don't just double the quantities. If, for example, you decide to cook for 4, double the meat and sauce/liquid quantities but only increase the spices, salt and sugar by 50%.

Calories & Measurements

The calories stated in each menu are the recipe ingredients only - anything you add to this will obviously increase the calories. Unless stated, calories for each meat dish have been based on 300g skinless chicken breasts. Other meats will increase calories.

Also feel free to substitute vegetables for meat if that's what you prefer, this will bring your calorie count down even more.

Cooking Tips

Adding salt, sugar and spice heat to your meals is a question of taste. Feel free to adjust the recipes to suit your own preferences.

Getting the right consistency for your curry is key. If you feel like it's not thick enough, leave to cook for a little longer with the lid off to thicken the sauce. Likewise, if it's too thick add some water to loosen things up during cooking. Also make sure your spices don't burn - this is really important.

As we've really cut down on the oil to make the meals skinny, you might find adding a drop of water to the pan when you are cooking the dry spices helps.

The final thing to mention is the use of sugar. If you find any of your curries have a slight bitterness to them, add some sugar to counteract. Use small amounts (½ tsp) a time to make sure you don't over do it.

The main thing is to be confident. Get started and you'll be cooking delicious takeaway style curries in no time.

Skinny Curry Base Mix
Makes 12 Servings

Ingredients:

1 tbsp sunflower oil
1 large onion chopped
2 carrots, sliced
1 tsp garlic powder
1 tsp cumin
1 tsp turmeric
1 tsp paprika
½ tsp garam masala
1 tsp ground coriander

½ tsp ground ginger
1 tsp salt
1 tsp sugar
2 tbsp tomato puree
1 400g/14oz can chopped tomatoes
600ml/2 ½ cups boiling water with 1 chicken stock cube

Method:

Gently sauté the onions and carrots in the oil for a few minutes. Add all the dried spices and tomato puree and cook for another minute or two. Add the stock, salt, sugar and chopped tomatoes, cover and leave to simmer very gently for 40 minutes. Blend until completely smooth and split into portions. You can keep chilled for a few days or freeze for a few months.

This skinny curry base sauce will form the base of most of the curries you make. You can divide or multiply the quantities to suit you. It makes sense to make up quite a big batch so you have it to hand whenever you have a curry craving.

Bhuna
Serves 2

427 CALORIES PER SERVING

Ingredients:

2 portions skinny curry base mix
300g/11oz lean meat, cubed
100g/3 ½ oz chopped vegetables
2 onions chopped
¼ tsp cardamom seeds
½ fenugreek seeds and ground ginger
1 tsp ground garlic
1 large tomato chopped

½ red or green pepper sliced
½ tsp each turmeric, chilli powder, ground coriander, cumin & garam masala
1 tbsp low fat natural yoghurt
1 tbsp tomato puree
½ tbsp lemon juice
½ tsp salt
1 tsp sugar
2 tsp sunflower oil

Method:

Brown the meat in a frying pan with the sunflower oil for a couple of minutes. Add the meat and meat juices into the slow cooker along with all the other ingredients except the yoghurt and lemon juice. Stir well, cover and leave to cook on high for 2-3 hours or low for 4-5 hours or until the meat is tender and cooked through. Stir through the yoghurt and lemon juice just before serving. If you find the curry is a little thick after/during cooking add a few drops of water and stir. Alternatively if it is not thick enough after cooking, remove the lid and leave to cook on high for 30-40 mins until you get the consistency you require.

Bhuna is a medium curry with a thick sauce which usually contains vegetables. Use whatever you have to hand, but a mix of carrots, cauliflower and peas is a good place to start.

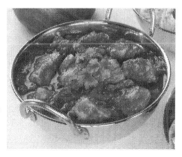

Jalfrezi
Serves 2

375
CALORIES
PER SERVING

Ingredients:

2 portions skinny curry base mix
300g/11oz lean meat cubed
1 medium onion thinly sliced
2 tsp sunflower oil
½ tsp each garlic powder, ground ginger, cumin, coriander & turmeric

1 red pepper sliced
1 tsp sugar
½ tsp salt
4 green chillies sliced
1 tsp chilli powder
4 fresh tomatoes, chopped
1 tbsp tomato puree/paste

Method:

Brown the meat in a frying pan with the sunflower oil for a couple of minutes. Add the meat and meat juices to the slow cooker along with all the other ingredients. Stir well, cover and leave to cook on high for 2-3 hours or low for 4-5 hours or until the meat is tender and cooked through. If you find the curry is a little thick after/during cooking add a few drops of water and stir. Alternatively if it is not thick enough, after cooking remove the lid and leave to cook on high for 30-40 mins until you get the consistency you require.

Jalfrezi should always contain green chillies and onions. It recently usurped Chicken Tikka Masala in a national poll as the UK's most popular curry.

Korma
Serves 2

Ingredients:

2 portions skinny curry base mix
300g/11oz lean meat cubed
1 tsp mild curry powder
¼ tsp ground ginger
½ tsp ground garlic, turmeric, garam masala, cumin
1 bay leaf
60ml/ ¼ cup low fat coconut milk

½ tsp sugar
½ tsp salt
Few drops natural yellow food colouring
2 tsp sunflower oil

Method:

Brown the meat in a frying pan with the sunflower oil for a couple of minutes. Add the meat and meat juices to the slow cooker along with all the other ingredients, except the coconut milk. Stir well, cover and leave to cook on high for 2-3 hours or low for 4-5 hours or until the meat is tender and cooked through. Stir through coconut milk and leave to warm for a few minutes. If you find the curry is a little thick after/during cooking, add a few drops of water and stir. Alternatively if it is not thick enough after cooking, remove the lid and leave to cook on high for 30-40 mins until you get the consistency you require.

A mild, yellow curry, Korma always contains almonds and/or coconut. This skinny version uses low fat coconut milk.

Madras
Serves 2

418 CALORIES PER SERVING

Ingredients:

2 portions skinny curry base mix
300g/11oz Lean meat
2 small onions finely chopped
1 tsp medium curry powder
½ tsp each of turmeric, fenugreek seeds, coriander, garlic powder, ground ginger, paprika & garam masala

3 fresh tomatoes chopped
1 tbsp tomato puree
1 ½ tsp chilli powder
½ tsp crushed cardamom seeds
½ tsp salt
1 tsp sugar
2 tsps lemon juice
2 tsp sunflower oil

Method:

Brown the meat in a frying pan with the sunflower oil for a couple of minutes. Add the meat and meat juices to the slow cooker along with all the other ingredients, except the lemon juice. Stir well, cover and leave to cook on high for 2-3 hours or low for 4-5 hours or until the meat is tender and cooked through. Stir through the lemon juice just before serving. If you find the curry is a little thick after/during cooking, add a few drops of water and stir. Alternatively if it is not thick enough after cooking, remove the lid and leave to cook on high for 30-40 mins until you get the consistency you require.

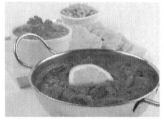

Known as the standard hot curry in the UK. Madras has a fiery reputation.

Rogan Josh
Serves 2

399
CALORIES
PER SERVING

Ingredients:

2 portions skinny curry base mix
300g/11oz lean cubed meat
1 tsp each garlic powder, ground ginger, cumin powder, garam masala
1 tsp sugar
½ tsp turmeric powder & ground cinnamon
2 tbsp ground almonds

2 tsp curry powder
1 tbsp paprika
½ tsp ground cinnamon
Pinch ground cloves
2 tbsp low fat Greek yoghurt
1 tbsp tomato puree/paste
3 chopped tomatoes
½ tsp salt
2 tsp sunflower oil

Method:

Brown the meat in a frying pan with the sunflower oil for a couple of minutes. Add the meat and meat juices to the slow cooker along with all the other ingredients, except the yoghurt. Stir well, cover and leave to cook on high for 2-3 hours or low for 4-5 hours or until the meat is tender and cooked through. Stir through the yoghurt just before serving. If you find the curry is a little thick after/during cooking, add a few drops of water and stir. Alternatively if it is not thick enough after cooking, remove the lid and leave to cook on high for 30-40 mins until you get the consistency you require.

Rogan Josh is an aromatic dish of Persian origin, popular in the Kashmir region.

Vindaloo
Serves 2

Ingredients:

2 portions skinny curry base mix
300g/11oz lean meat
2 tsp hot chilli powder (or to your taste)
1 tbsp white wine vinegar
1 tsp turmeric, paprika, garlic, cumin, garam masala

1 tsp chilli powder
4 fresh tomatoes, chopped
1 tbsp tomato puree
1 onion sliced
1 tbsp tomato puree
1 tsp sugar
½ tsp salt
2 tsp sunflower oil

Method:

Brown the meat in a frying pan with the sunflower oil for a couple of minutes. Add the meat and meat juices to the slow cooker along with all the other ingredients. Stir well, cover and leave to cook on high for 2-3 hours or low for 4-5 hours or until the meat is tender and cooked through. If you find the curry is a little thick after/during cooking, add a few drops of water and stir. Alternatively if it is not thick enough after cooking, remove the lid and leave to cook on high for 30-40 mins until you get the consistency you require.

Vindaloo is all about the heat! The version here is reasonably hot but feel free to adjust to your taste.

CONVERSION CHART: DRY INGREDIENTS

Metric	Imperial
7g	¼ oz
15g	½ oz
20g	¾ oz
25g	1 oz
40g	1½oz
50g	2oz
60g	2½oz
75g	3oz
100g	3½oz
125g	4oz
140g	4½oz
150g	5oz
165g	5½oz
175g	6oz
200g	7oz
225g	8oz
250g	9oz
275g	10oz
300g	11oz
350g	12oz
375g	13oz
400g	14oz

Metric	Imperial
425g	15oz
450g	1lb
500g	1lb 2oz
550g	1¼lb
600g	1lb 5oz
650g	1lb 7oz
675g	1½lb
700g	1lb 9oz
750g	1lb 11oz
800g	1¾lb
900g	2lb
1kg	2¼lb
1.1kg	2½lb
1.25kg	2¾lb
1.35kg	3lb
1.5kg	3lb 6oz
1.8kg	4lb
2kg	4½lb
2.25kg	5lb
2.5kg	5½lb
2.75kg	6lb

CONVERSION CHART: LIQUID MEASURES

Metric	Imperial	US
25ml	1fl oz	
60ml	2fl oz	¼ cup
75ml	2½ fl oz	
100ml	3½fl oz	
120ml	4fl oz	½ cup
150ml	5fl oz	
175ml	6fl oz	
200ml	7fl oz	
250ml	8½ fl oz	1 cup
300ml	10½ fl oz	
360ml	12½ fl oz	
400ml	14fl oz	
450ml	15½ fl oz	
600ml	1 pint	
750ml	1¼ pint	3 cups
1 litre	1½ pints	4 cups

🍎 **CookNation**

Other
COOKNATION
TITLES

If you enjoyed 'The Skinny Slow Cooker Recipe Book' we'd really appreciate your feedback. Reviews help others decide if this is the right book for them so a moment of your time would be appreciated.

Thank you.

You may also be interested in other '**Skinny**' titles in the CookNation series. You can find all the following great titles by searching under '**CookNation**'.

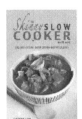

The Skinny Slow Cooker Recipe Book

Delicious Recipes Under 300, 400 And 500 Calories.

Paperback / eBook

More Skinny Slow Cooker Recipes

75 More Delicious Recipes Under 300, 400 & 500 Calories.

Paperback / eBook

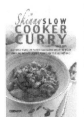

The Skinny Slow Cooker Curry Recipe Book

Low Calorie Curries From Around The World

Paperback / eBook

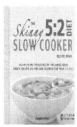

The Skinny Slow Cooker Soup Recipe Book

Simple, Healthy & Delicious Low Calorie Soup Recipes For Your Slow Cooker. All Under 100, 200 & 300 Calories.

Paperback / eBook

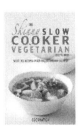

The Skinny Slow Cooker Vegetarian Recipe Book

40 Delicious Recipes Under 200, 300 And 400 Calories.

Paperback / eBook

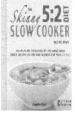

The Skinny 5:2 Slow Cooker Recipe Book

Skinny Slow Cooker Recipe And Menu Ideas Under 100, 200, 300 & 400 Calories For Your 5:2 Diet.

Paperback / eBook

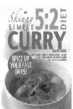

The Skinny 5:2 Curry Recipe Book

Spice Up Your Fast Days With Simple Low Calorie Curries, Snacks, Soups, Salads & Sides Under 200, 300 & 400 Calories

Paperback / eBook

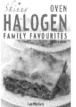

The Skinny Halogen Oven Family Favourites Recipe Book

Healthy, Low Calorie Family Meal-Time Halogen Oven Recipes Under 300, 400 and 500 Calories

Paperback / eBook

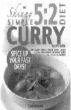

Skinny Halogen Oven Cooking For One

Single Serving, Healthy, Low Calorie Halogen Oven Recipes Under 200, 300 and 400 Calories

Paperback / eBook

Skinny Winter Warmers Recipe Book

Soups, Stews, Casseroles & One Pot Meals Under 300, 400 & 500 Calories.

Paperback / eBook

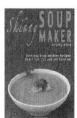

The Skinny Soup Maker Recipe Book

Delicious Low Calorie, Healthy and Simple Soup Recipes Under 100, 200 and 300 Calories. Perfect For Any Diet and Weight Loss Plan.

Paperback / eBook

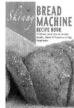

The Skinny Bread Machine Recipe Book

70 Simple, Lower Calorie, Healthy Breads...Baked To Perfection In Your Bread Maker.

Paperback / eBook

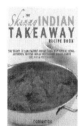

The Skinny Indian Takeaway Recipe Book

Authentic British Indian Restaurant Dishes Under 300, 400 And 500 Calories. The Secret To Low Calorie Indian Takeaway Food At Home

Paperback / eBook

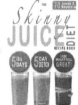
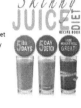

The Skinny Juice Diet Recipe Book

5lbs, 5 Days. The Ultimate Kick-Start Diet and Detox Plan to Lose Weight & Feel Great!

Paperback / eBook

Available only on eBook

The Skinny 5:2 Diet Recipe Book Collection

All The 5:2 Fast Diet Recipes You'll Ever Need. All Under 100, 200, 300, 400 And 500 Calories

eBook

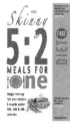

The Skinny 5:2 Fast Diet Meals For One

Single Serving Fast Day Recipes & Snacks Under 100, 200 & 300 Calories

Paperback / eBook

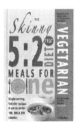

The Skinny 5:2 Fast Diet Vegetarian Meals For One

Single Serving Fast Day Recipes & Snacks Under 100, 200 & 300 Calories

Paperback / eBook

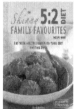

The Skinny 5:2 Fast Diet Family Favourites Recipe Book

Eat With All The Family On Your Diet Fasting Days

Paperback / eBook

Available only on eBook

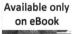

The Skinny 5:2 Fast Diet Family Favorites Recipe Book *U.S.A. EDITION*

Dine With All The Family On Your Diet Fasting Days

Paperback / eBook

The Skinny 5:2 Diet Chicken Dishes Recipe Book

Delicious Low Calorie Chicken Dishes Under 300, 400 & 500 Calories

Paperback / eBook

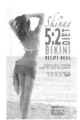

The Skinny 5:2 Bikini Diet Recipe Book

Recipes & Meal Planners Under 100, 200 & 300 Calories. Get Ready For Summer & Lose Weight...FAST!

Paperback / eBook

Available only on eBook

The Paleo Diet For Beginners Slow Cooker Recipe Book

Gluten Free, Everyday Essential Slow Cooker Paleo Recipes For Beginners

eBook

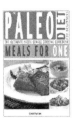

The Paleo Diet For Beginners Meals For One

The Ultimate Paleo Single Serving Cookbook

Paperback / eBook

Available only on eBook

The Paleo Diet For Beginners Holidays

Thanksgiving, Christmas & New Year Paleo Friendly Recipes

eBook

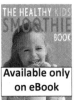

Available only on eBook

The Healthy Kids Smoothie Book

40 Delicious Goodness In A Glass Recipes for Happy Kids.

eBook

The Skinny Slow Cooker Summer Recipe Book

Fresh & Seasonal Summer Recipes For Your Slow Cooker. All Under 300, 400 And 500 Calories.

Paperback / eBook

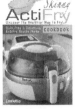

The Skinny ActiFry Cookbook

Guilt-free and Delicious ActiFry Recipe Ideas: Discover The Healthier Way to Fry!

Paperback / eBook

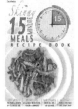

The Skinny 15 Minute Meals Recipe Book

Delicious, Nutritious & Super-Fast Meals in 15 Minutes Or Less. All Under 300, 400 & 500 Calories.

Paperback / eBook

The Skinny Mediterranean Recipe Book

Simple, Healthy & Delicious Low Calorie Mediterranean Diet Dishes. All Under 200, 300 & 400 Calories.

Paperback / eBook

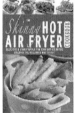

The Skinny Hot Air Fryer Cookbook

Delicious & Simple Meals For Your Hot Air Fryer: Discover The Healthier Way To Fry.

Paperback / eBook

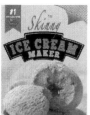

The Skinny Ice Cream Maker

Delicious Lower Fat, Lower Calorie Ice Cream, Frozen Yogurt & Sorbet Recipes For Your Ice Cream Maker

Paperback / eBook

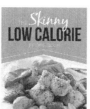

The Skinny Low Calorie Recipe Book

Great Tasting, Simple & Healthy Meals Under 300, 400 & 500 Calories. Perfect For Any Calorie Controlled Diet.

Paperback / eBook

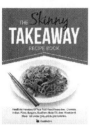

The Skinny Takeaway Recipe Book

Healthier Versions Of Your Fast Food Favourites: Chinese, Indian, Pizza, Burgers, Southern Style Chicken, Mexican & More. All Under 300, 400 & 500 Calories

Paperback / eBook

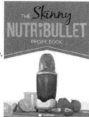

The Skinny Nutribullet Recipe Book

80+ Delicious & Nutritious Healthy Smoothie Recipes. Burn Fat, Lose Weight and Feel Great!

Paperback / eBook

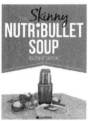

The Skinny Nutribullet Soup Recipe Book

Delicious, Quick & Easy, Single Serving Soups & Pasta Sauces For Your Nutribullet. All Under 100, 200, 300 & 400 Calories.

Paperback / eBook

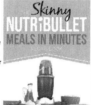

The Skinny Nutribullet Meals In Minutes Recipe Book

Quick & Easy, Single Serving Suppers, Snacks, Sauces, Salad Dressings & More. All Under 300, 400 & 500 Calories.

Paperback / eBook

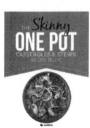

The Skinny One-Pot Recipe book

Simple & Delicious, One-Pot Meals. All Under 300, 400 & 500 Calories

Paperback / eBook

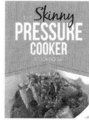

The Skinny Pressure Cooker Cookbook

USA ONLY

Low Calorie, Healthy & Delicious Meals, Sides & Desserts. All Under 300, 400 & 500 Calories.

Paperback / eBook

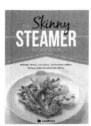

The Skinny Steamer Recipe Book

Delicious, Healthy, Low Calorie, Low Fat Steam Cooking Recipes Under 300, 400 & 500 Calories

Paperback / eBook

23306146R00063

Printed in Poland
by Amazon Fulfillment
Poland Sp. z o.o., Wrocław